anita bean's

six week workout

FAB ABS

Before starting this or any other exercise programme, you should check with your doctor if you have any health problems, are taking medication, are recovering from an injury or illness or if you haven't taken exercise for over a year.

While the advice and information in this book is believed to be accurate and up to date, it is advisory only and should not be used as an alternative to seeking specialist medical advice. The author and publishers cannot be held responsible for any injury sustained while following the exercises or using the information contained in this book, which are taken entirely at the reader's own risk.

Published in 2005 by A & C Black Publishers Ltd
37 Soho Square, London W1D 3QZ
www.acblack.com

Copyright © 2005 by Anita Bean

ISBN 0 7136 7197 1

A CIP record for this book is available from the British Library.

Note: While every effort has been made to ensure that the content of this book is as technically accurate and as sound as possible, neither the author nor the publisher can accept responsibility for any injury or loss sustained as a result of the use of this material.

A & C Black uses paper produced with elemental chlorine-free pulp, harvested from managed sustainable forests.

Acknowledgements
Cover photography courtesy of Zefa
Illustrations by James Wakelin
Text photography by Grant Pritchard

Printed and bound in Singapore by Tien Wah Press (Pte) Ltd

contents

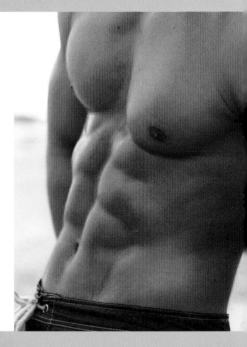

acknowledgements

Many thanks to my husband Simon, and daughters Chloe and Lucy, for all their support. A big thank you to photographer Grant Pritchard, personal trainer Steve Tunstall (www.stpersonaltraining.co.uk) for demonstrating the exercises, and my editors at A & C Black, Claire Dunn and Hannah McEwen.

Photos were shot on location at Holmes Place, Epsom.

introduction

What's the first thing you notice about a fit physique on the beach or by the pool? Great costume? Super tan? No – the chances are you'll be struck by those fabulous abs. They're sexy, right? And they're the trademark of a fit body.

Let's be honest: a lean midsection is on top of everyone's 'most wanted' list. It's not only attractive, but it also tells the world that you look after your body. Unlike any other body part, it speaks volumes about your lifestyle. It says that you care about what you look like, you watch what you eat, and you work out hard. You see, a toned midsection is a mission statement.

When your abs are in great shape, you look taller, smarter and more confident. Your posture improves as strong abs ensure your shoulders, hips and back are in proper alignment, and you look more relaxed. There's no bulge to disguise under a long sweater. There's no discomfort when you do up your belt. When your abs are well-toned you can wear pretty much what you like – with no fear of popping a button.

But strong abs are also important for the prevention of lower back problems. These muscles stabilise your pelvis and torso, which, in turn, support your back.

So, how do you get fab abs?

Unlike building up the chest or arms – essentially the product of lifting heavy weights – a lean midsection is the result of super-smart training and intelligent eating.

And that's precisely what this book is about. It's a six-week workout that focuses on your abs. It's a three-pronged attack that incorporates the most effective abdominal exercises ever; cardiovascular exercise for maximum fat-burning; and a delicious eating plan guaranteed to rev your metabolism and strip fat.

The truth of the matter is everyone has a six-pack. It's just that it's hidden by a layer of fat. In six weeks you'll have a midsection to be proud of. And, who knows, it may well be you who'll be turning a few heads on the beach this year.

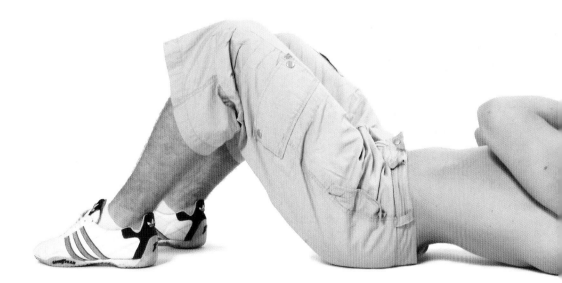

countdown

The ab workouts in this book take less than NINE MINUTES. Yes, you read that right. All they require is nine minutes of your time every other day – that's less time than it takes to eat a sandwich! During this time, you'll be performing a circuit of exercises that specifically target your abs. And each week you'll change your workout to challenge your abs further and – importantly – keep boredom at bay.

In addition, you'll include a minimum of 20 minutes of cardiovascular exercise five times a week. This will burn fat and shift your metabolism into a higher gear. Together with a smart eating plan, you'll be fast-tracking towards your best abs ever. So what are you waiting for?

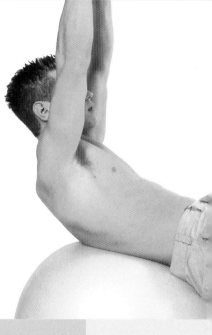

your abs

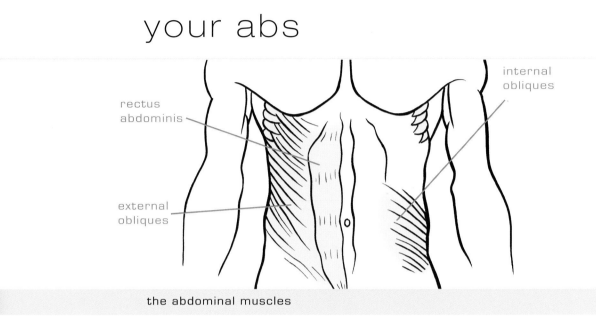

rectus
abdominis

external
obliques

internal
obliques

the abdominal muscles

Your abs are comprised of four separate muscles. These muscles support and help move the torso:

1. The **rectus abdominis** (the 'six-pack' muscle), the long slender muscle that runs vertically down your abdomen from your lower ribs to your pubic bone. It flexes the torso so the ribcage moves towards the pelvis.

2. The **external obliques**, which cover the front and side of your abdomen and run diagonally from the lower ribs to the pelvis to form a 'V' shape. They bend the torso sideways and rotate it to the opposite side when flexing forwards.

3. The **internal obliques**, directly underneath the external obliques but running in the opposite direction to form an inverted 'V' shape. They help the rectus abdominis bend the torso forwards, as well as rotating it to the same side to which they are attached.

4. The **transverse abdominis (TVA)**, a flat sheath of muscle lying underneath the rectus abdominis, running across the torso. It originates in the lower spine, and wraps around and attaches to the ribs, abdominals and pelvis. It acts as a muscular girdle to hold in your internal organs.

core training

To get truly fab abs, you need a strong torso or 'core'. This six-week workout focuses on developing core stability and strength by using proven principles of core training.

what is core training?

Core training is based on the idea that by training the muscles surrounding the torso, pelvis and spine – in particular the TVA and the lumbar multifidus in the lower back – you can increase stability throughout your entire body. These trunk muscles act as a natural girdle, stabilising your pelvis and supporting your torso. All movement starts from the TVA – or at least it should. In many cases, due to inactive lifestyles, people no longer have control over this muscle and so develop bad posture, back problems and poor movement quality.

what are the benefits of core training?

Traditional exercises have little effect on core strength as they do not work the trunk stabilisers. But training your core, and learning how to 'switch on' your TVA, helps stabilise your pelvis, and builds better balance and posture by correctly aligning your body. It also helps improve performance in other sports, prevent injury, and strengthen a weak lower back – as well as tone a flabby midsection. When you work to strengthen and stabilise your core, you strengthen your body's power base.

how can you do it?

There are many exercises that improve core stability – Pilates is one of the best-known stability programmes. Others involve exercising from an unstable base such as an exercise ball. This places a higher demand on the deep muscles in the core, as well as on your motor control system, because you constantly have to stabilise yourself as the ball rolls around.

The six-week workout in this book includes exercises with an exercise ball to work your core muscles. Throughout, there is a major focus on developing core strength, balance and good posture.

good posture

To find your **neutral posture**, where your joints are aligned correctly to each other, stand with your feet hip-width apart, knees relaxed. Let your shoulders drop down and away from your ears. Lengthen your spine and neck – imagine a string attached to the top of your head, pulling you up to the ceiling. Contract your abdominal muscles, drawing your navel in towards your spine. Adjust the tilt of your pelvis so that it is in a neutral position. You should be able to draw a line vertically from your shoulders to your hips and feet.

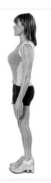

exercise tips

think ribs and hips

The function of the abs is to draw the hips and ribcage together in a crunching movement. So, for every exercise, picture your ribcage and pelvis pulling together. Don't worry about how far you are moving – it's the direction of movement that is most important.

go for slow mo

Do each movement in a slow and controlled manner. This increases the intensity of the contraction and minimises injury risk. One of the most common errors is performing the movements too quickly in the belief it will melt fat away. This is not true – fast movements generate excess momentum and reduce the effectiveness of the exercise.

get s-shaped

Maintain a neutral alignment of the spine at all times by keeping the natural 'S' contour. Although your spine flexes during many of the exercises, keep your neck, head and shoulders in alignment. Don't press your chin into your chest – imagine you are holding an apple under your chin. This neutral position distributes the load more evenly and minimises stress to the vertebrae and discs of the spine.

go all the way

Aim to perform each exercise with a full range of movement, really squeezing the muscles.

breathe right

Breathe in during the relaxation (easier) part of the movement and exhale during the contraction (harder) part of the movement.

work your abs every other day

Training your abs every other day is sufficient. Working them more frequently won't necessarily produce better results, and risks over-training and injury. If your abs are still sore, it's too soon to train them again.

rep rule

The number of repetitions you can manage depends on how hard you squeeze your abs at the top of each movement. It's better to perform slower, intense movements with good control, holding each contraction for a count of two, than rushing to perform more reps. Use the recommended rep ranges in the workouts as a guide. If you can do more, try slowing the movement to make the reps harder. When it starts to hurt (not to be confused with actual pain), move on to the next exercise.

variety is key

You should always include a variety of abdominal exercises in your routine to target each area and to prevent your muscles from becoming too used to the same exercises. Do some crunch-type movements for the upper region, reverse crunch-type movements for the lower region, and movements with a slight twisting motion for the obliques. The six workouts in this book make sure you work the entire abdominal region.

Q & A - *frequently asked questions*

I always thought that sit-ups were one of the best exercises for the abs. Is this true?

The traditional feet-restrained sit-up is not recommended in this six-week workout as it can put stress on the lower back and aggravate back pain. This is because the psoas muscle – a hip flexor, which attaches to the fourth and fifth lumbar vertebrae – is involved in the movement (even if your knees are bent). When you bring your chest towards your hips from a lying position, the hip flexors initially do most of the work. Only in the last part of the movement do the abdominals contract. So, not only is the movement largely ineffective for the abs, it can also put stress on the lower back. Keep your knees slightly bent and your feet unsecured to minimise hip flexor involvement when doing abdominal exercises.

Can abdominal training help or hinder back problems?

Weak abdominals are often associated with back problems. Overstretched, slack muscles, combined with tight hip flexors (connecting the thigh bone to the lower vertebrae), can cause the pelvis to tilt forwards (lordosis). This creates an excessive arch in the lower back and potential back pain. Strong abdominals support and stabilise the pelvis and lower back. Strengthening these muscles (and stretching the hip flexors) will eliminate excessive arching in the lower back, give good posture and minimise potential back problems.

Will I get a better workout with one of those ab machines I've seen advertised?

While there's nothing wrong with most ab machines – they are helpful initially for ensuring your body is positioned correctly – you can get great (if not better) results from basic exercises that require nothing more than the floor and an exercise ball. Use strict form and good control, follow the exercise tips on pages 4–5 and save your money!

Why have some people got a six-pack even though they don't train their abs?

A fortunate few have visible abs despite doing no direct abs training. This is due to their exceptionally low level of body fat, most likely the result of general sport training. The truth of the matter is we all have a six-pack; the problem is the layer of fat covering it up. For the abs to become visible, men need to reduce their body fat level below about 12 per cent and women below 18 per cent – levels lower than those of the general population. Abdominal exercises are not a direct ticket to a six-pack, although they will tone and shape your abs. You also need to remove the fat through exercise and diet (see pages 44–51 and 62–80).

Despite doing lots of abdominal exercises, my stomach still sticks out. How can I get a flat stomach?

This is a common problem. A protruding belly is usually the combined result of poor posture, performing abdominal exercises such as crunches incorrectly and neglecting to train your transverse abdominis (TVA), the flat sheet of muscle lying beneath your six-pack muscle. To rectify this, gently draw your belly button towards your spine during all abdominal exercises, flattening rather than crunching up your midsection. Do specific exercises for your TVA, such as the plank (see page 19), pelvic tilt (see page 11), lying alternate leg extensions (see page 24), and the scissor kick (see page 38). Include ab exercises on an exercise ball to work the core muscles and improve your posture. Even when you're not exercising – when you're sitting, standing or walking – try to keep your hips 'neutral' by gently tightening your TVA muscle.

I work out regularly but can't seem to get rid of my love handles. Any ideas?

Those stubborn love handles are basically excess fat. It's not possible to burn fat selectively from this or any part of your body. But you can reduce your overall body fat and rev your metabolism by including regular cardiovascular (CV) exercise in your programme and watching your calorie intake. Try the six-week CV workout on pages 44–51, follow the diet on pages 62–80 and watch those love handles melt away.

What results can I realistically expect to see in just six weeks?

This six-week workout is designed to kick-start good eating and training habits. How quickly you will see a visible change depends on your initial ab strength and fat levels. If you already work out and carry relatively little fat, you can expect to get visible abs in six weeks with this workout. But whatever your starting level, you will notice a significant improvement in the appearance and tone of your midsection in six weeks. Expect to lose up to 6 kg (13 lb) of fat (depending on your initial weight and goal) in this time. If you need to lose more, continue with this programme until you reach your goal.

exercises

This six-week abs programme is an intense workout designed to get fast results. It is divided into six workouts, which increase in difficulty as the weeks progress. All the workouts devote time to each portion of the abdominal musculature – the upper area, the obliques and the lower area – with a variety of effective exercises. There is a central focus on core strength throughout – the muscles surrounding your torso, pelvis and spine – to increase the strength and stability of your whole body. This will develop good posture, proper alignment of the hips and – best of all – a gorgeous flat stomach.

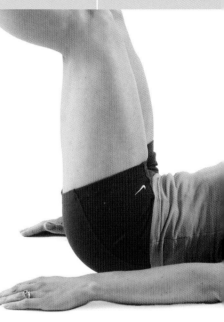

You can do your abs workouts either at the end of your regular workout (say, at the gym or after playing sport) or at any other time of day that fits into your schedule. The important thing is to do it three times a week. As it only takes nine minutes, that's not too much to ask, is it?

workout rules

■ Each workout should be completed three times a week.

■ Rest for at least one day between workouts.

■ Aim to complete the suggested repetitions (reps) – otherwise just do as many as you can.

■ If you experience discomfort, rest, then continue the workout.

■ Each workout should take about nine minutes to complete.

■ If you complete the workout in under nine minutes, try slowing down your movements, concentrating on squeezing your muscles and holding each contraction a little longer.

■ If you find any of the exercises too difficult, adapt the movement so that it feels easier or substitute a similar exercise that you are more familiar with until you develop enough strength.

■ Focus on each movement – don't rush any exercise.

■ Visualise your performance and your desired result – cut out a photo and stick it on your wall or fridge to keep you motivated.

week 1

the goal

The goal of the first week is to develop a good base of abdominal strength and introduce you to a repertoire of exercises that work each area of the abdominal region.

■ Perform all the exercises listed below (this is one circuit), then repeat the circuit one more time.

■ Rest for 15 seconds between exercises; rest for 30 seconds after you finish a circuit.

■ You should complete the workout in no more than nine minutes.

■ Perform each repetition with good technique (see exercise tips, pages 4–5).

exercise	reps
Pelvic tilt	15–20
Twisting exercise	
ball crunch	10–12
Side bridge	5
Crunch	12–20

pelvic tilt

target muscles: rectus abdominis (mainly lower), transverse abdominis

starting position

1. Lie on your back with your hands by your sides. Bend your knees and place your feet flat on the floor. Make sure your back is in its natural arch.

movement

1. Now flatten out your lower back, pressing the small of your back into the floor. Your hips should roll automatically towards your chest. Hold for 5 seconds then return to the starting position.

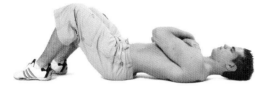 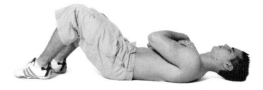

TIP

This movement is quite subtle and small – just go far enough to feel your abs contracting before holding.

twisting exercise ball crunch

target muscles: internal and external obliques, rectus abdominis

starting position

1. Sit on top of an exercise ball, feet on the floor. Slide forwards, rolling the ball under your bottom until your lower back is centred on top of the ball.

2. Place your hands by the sides of your head.

movement

1. Slowly raise your upper body, rotating one elbow towards the opposite knee.

2. Pause briefly as you contract your obliques, then return to the starting position, rotating your body back to its original position.

3. Repeat to the opposite side.

TIPS

- Lead with your shoulder rather than your elbow.

- Don't pull on your head – use your abs and obliques to raise and rotate your torso.

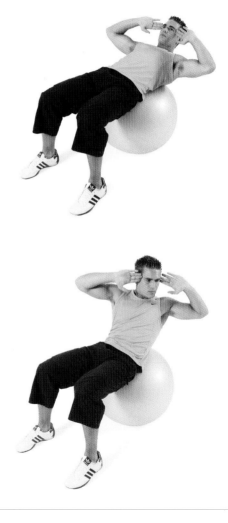

side bridge

target muscles: obliques, transverse abdominis

starting position

1. Lie on your right side, using your elbow to prop up your body. Your elbow should be under your shoulder.
2. Your legs should be straight.

movement

1. Lift your hips so that only your right forearm and right ankle are in contact with the floor.
2. Your body should be in a straight line. Keep your spine long and in neutral alignment.
3. Hold for 5–10 seconds, then slowly lower back to the start position. Do five reps, then switch sides and do five more reps.

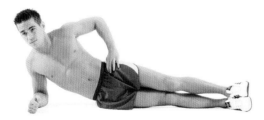

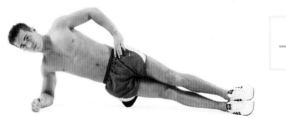

TIPS

- Lift your hips as high as possible without rolling forwards or backwards.
- Keep your hips stacked on top of each other.
- Keep your neck neutral and in line with your spine.

Make it harder: Support your upper body on your hand instead of your forearm. You can raise your left (top) arm to the ceiling.

crunch

target muscles: rectus abdominis (mainly upper part)

starting position

1. Lie flat on your back, either on the floor or on an abdominal bench, with your knees bent over your hips and your ankles touching. If you are on the floor, you can rest your feet on a bench with your knees bent at 90 degrees.
2. Place your hands lightly by the sides of your head or across your chest.
3. Press your lower back to the floor or bench.

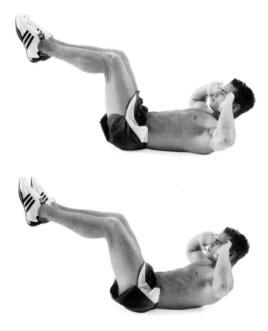

movement

1. Use your abdominal strength to raise your head and shoulders from the floor or bench. You should only come up about 10 cm and your lower back should remain on the floor.
2. Hold this contracted position for a count of two.
3. Let your body uncurl slowly back to the starting position.

Make it easier: Place your feet flat on the floor, knees bent at about 60 degrees. Or cross your arms over your chest.

Make it harder: Perform the movement with your legs straight up in the air. With your arms in front of you, curl up, reaching towards your toes, then slowly lower yourself back down.

TIPS
- Focus on moving your ribs towards your hips.
- Don't pull your head with your hands – keep your elbows out and relaxed.
- Exhale as you contract your abdominals.

week 2

the goal

Now you've become familiar with the major abdominal exercises and started to develop good abdominal control, you are ready to get to grips with some new exercises that will improve your core strength. Listen to your body throughout, aiming to perform each movement through the full range of motion.

■ Perform all the exercises listed below (this is one circuit), then repeat the circuit one more time.

■ Rest for 15 seconds between exercises; rest for 30 seconds after you finish a circuit.

■ You should complete the workout in no more than nine minutes.

■ Perform each repetition with good technique (see exercise tips, pages 4–5).

exercise	reps
Exercise ball crunch	12 – 15
Twisting crunch	10 – 12
Exercise ball pull-in	10
Plank	1

WOODMILL HIGH SCHOOL

exercise ball crunch

target muscles: rectus abdominis (mainly upper portion), transverse abdominis

starting position

1. Sit on top of an exercise ball, feet on the floor. Slide forwards, rolling the ball under your bottom until your lower back is centred on top of the ball.

2. Cross your arms over your chest or, to make the exercise harder, place your hands by the sides of your head.

movement

1. Making sure that you move only your upper body and that your lower back remains in contact with the ball, slowly raise your torso.

2. Hold the position for a count of two, then lower yourself back to the starting position.

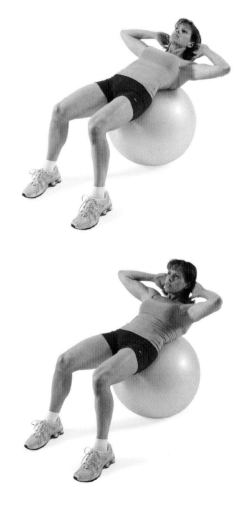

TIPS

• Keep the movement controlled when you lower yourself back down.

• Don't let your upper body arch backwards or your head flop back over the ball.

• To make the movement harder, bring your whole body higher up on to the top of the ball.

twisting crunch

target muscles: internal and external obliques, rectus abdominis

starting position

1. Lie on your back with your knees bent and feet either in the air or flat on the floor.
2. Place your hands by the side of your head.

movement

1. Lift your right shoulder diagonally, aiming it towards your left knee.
2. Hold for two counts, then slowly return to your starting position.
3. After completing the required number of repetitions, repeat the exercise on the other side.

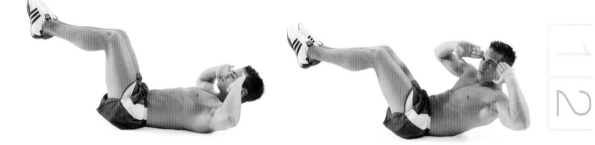

TIPS

- Imagine your ribcage rotating to the side as you curl up.
- Lead with your shoulder rather than your elbow.
- Make sure you lower your upper body slowly back to the floor.
- Do not twist your head, only your torso.
- Exhale as you contract your abdominals.

Make it harder: As you curl up, simultaneously bring your left knee in towards your left shoulder.

exercise ball pull-in

target muscles: rectus abdominis, transverse abdominis

starting position

1. Get into a push-up position, placing the lower part of your shins on top of an exercise ball.
2. Your head, back, hips and knees should be in a straight line.

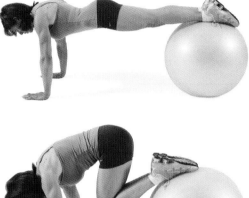

movement

1. Slowly pull your knees in towards your chest, allowing the ball to roll forwards under your ankles.
2. Hold for a moment with your abs contracted. Return to the start position by straightening your legs and rolling the ball away from your body.

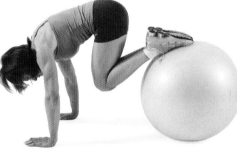

TIPS

- Try tucking your chin into your chest during the movement.
- Keep your back as straight as possible.

plank

target muscles: rectus abdominis, transverse abdominis

starting position

1. Lie face down with your hips and legs in contact with the floor and your upper body raised and supported on your forearms.
2. Your elbows should be directly under your shoulders by the sides of your body, palms down.

movement

1. Lift your hips so that only your forearms and toes are on the floor. Keep your spine in neutral alignment – your head, back, hips and ankles should be in a straight line.
2. Hold for 60–120 seconds, then slowly lower yourself back to the starting position.

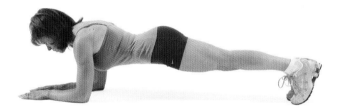

TIPS

- Keep your abs held in during the movement to protect your back.
- Check your neck, torso and legs are in a straight line.
- Make sure you don't let your bottom lift higher than your shoulders.
- Keep your shoulders pulled down and try to lengthen the distance between your shoulders and ears.

week 3

the goal

By week 3, you are ready to step up the intensity. Reduce the amount of rest between exercises to just 5–10 seconds, just long enough to move into the starting position of the next movement. Your abdominals will continue to be challenged by new exercises that work them in a variety of movement planes.

■ Perform all the exercises listed below (this is one circuit), then repeat the circuit one more time.

■ Rest for 5–10 seconds between exercises; rest for 30 seconds after you finish a circuit.

■ You should complete the workout in no more than nine minutes.

■ Perform each repetition with good technique (see exercise tips, pages 4–5).

exercise	reps
Reverse crunch	10 – 12
Exercise ball jackknife	10 – 12
Side crunch	10
Lying alternate leg extensions	12 – 15

reverse crunch

target muscles: rectus abdominis (mainly lower part)

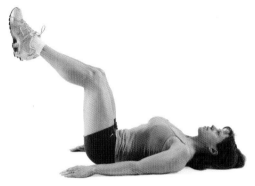

starting position

1. Lie flat on your back on the floor or on a bench with your knees bent over your hips and your ankles touching (as for crunches).

2. Place your arms alongside your body, palms flat on the floor, or hold on to the sides of the bench.

3. Press your lower back to the floor or bench.

movement

1. Slowly curl your hips off the floor, aiming your knees towards your chest. Your hips should rise no more than 10 cm.

2. Hold for a count of two.

3. Slowly lower your hips to the starting position, maintaining constant tension in your abdominals.

Make it harder: Try performing this exercise on an incline board.

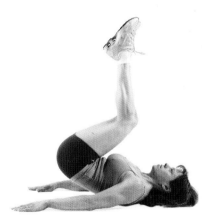

TIPS

• This should be a controlled, deliberate movement. Do not jerk, swing or bounce your hips off the floor; curl one vertebra up at a time.

• Do not allow your abdominals to relax at the top of the movement or while you are uncurling.

• Exhale as you contract your abdominals.

exercise ball jackknife

target muscles: rectus abdominis, transverse abdominis

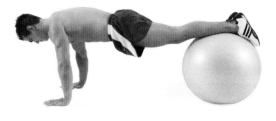

starting position

1. Get into a push-up position, resting the lower part of your shins on top of an exercise ball.
2. Make sure your arms, back and legs are straight.

movement

1. Slowly pull your lower body in towards your hands, allowing the ball to roll forwards and raising your hips as high as you can.
2. Pause, contracting your abs hard, then roll the ball back to the start position.

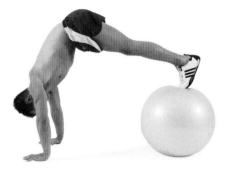

TIPS

- This exercise requires considerable core strength and upper body strength so practise the movement with a spotter first.
- Keep the movement smooth and controlled.
- Roll the ball in as close to your hands as possible and tuck your chin in – your torso should be almost vertical.

side crunch

target muscles: internal and external obliques, rectus abdominis

starting position

1. Lie on the floor or on an abdominal bench on your side with your knees slightly bent.

2. Place your top arm behind your head.

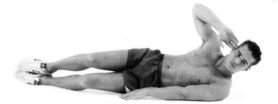

movement

1. Slowly exhale as you raise your head and shoulders a short distance off the floor or bench, aiming your ribs towards your top hip.

2. Hold for a count of two, then breathe in as you return to the starting position.

3. Repeat for the required number of repetitions, then perform the exercise on your other side.

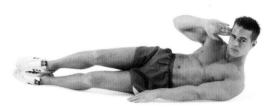

TIPS

• Aim to reduce the space between your ribs and hips.

• Don't worry if you can't reach up very far – concentrate on feeling the movement.

• Keep your head in line with your body – don't jerk it upwards.

lying alternate leg extensions

target muscles: rectus abdominis (mainly lower), transverse abdominis

starting position

1. Lie on your back with your hands lightly supporting your head.

2. Raise your head and shoulders slightly off the floor, keeping your head in alignment with your body. Lift your legs so that your thighs are at right angles to the floor and your lower legs are parallel, i.e. your knees and hips each make an angle of 90 degrees.

movement

1. Slowly extend your right leg away from your body so that it is almost parallel to the floor but not quite touching. Focus on keeping your spine in a neutral position (don't let it arch) and your pelvis level.

2. Bring your right leg back slowly to the starting position, again ensuring your spine remains neutral. Repeat with the left leg.

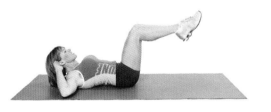
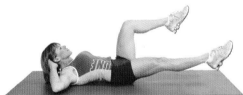

TIP

To make the exercise easier, keep the extended leg fairly high off the floor. As you get stronger, you can extend it at a lower angle.

week 4

the goal

To challenge your abdominal muscles further, you will now perform the exercises as two 'supersets'. Do the first exercise immediately followed by the second exercise. Rest for 30 seconds before repeating the superset

■ Perform the two exercises in the first superset. Rest for 30 seconds then repeat one more time.

■ Next, perform the second superset in the same manner, resting for 30 seconds between sets.

■ You should complete the workout in no more than nine minutes.

■ Perform each repetition with good technique (see exercise tips, pages 4–5).

exercise	sets	reps
Superset 1		
Hip thrust	2	12 – 15
Pullover crunch on exercise ball	2	12 – 20
Superset 2		
Hanging leg raise	2	10 – 12
Lateral exercise ball crunch	2	12 – 15

hip thrust

target muscles: rectus abdominis (mainly lower part), transverse abdominis

starting position

1. Lie flat on your back with your arms on the floor alongside your body, palms down.
2. Lift your legs at a right angle to the floor. They should be straight.

movement

1. Use your abs to lift your hips only a few centimetres off the floor, aiming your heels towards the ceiling.
2. Hold for a count of two.
3. Slowly lower your hips to the starting position, maintaining constant tension in your abdominals.

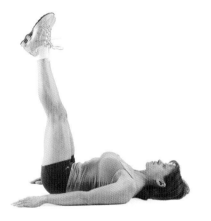

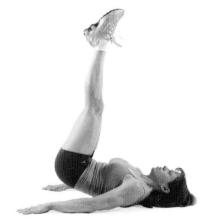

TIPS

- The range of motion is very limited – your hips should be raised no more than 10 cm.
- Keep the movement slow and controlled – do not jerk, swing or bounce your hips off the floor.

Make it easier: Bend your knees at about 60 degrees.

pullover crunch on exercise ball

target muscles: rectus abdominis (mainly upper portion), transverse abdominis

starting position

1. Sit on top of an exercise ball, feet on the floor. Slide forwards, rolling the ball under your bottom until your lower back is centred on top of the ball.
2. Hold a weight plate or dumbbell with both hands and extend your arms overhead.

movement

1. Slowly roll your shoulders towards your hips while keeping your arms extended overhead.
2. Hold the position for a count of two, then lower yourself back to the starting position.

TIP

Start by performing this exercise without a weight, then gradually add a 2.5 or 5 kg weight as you get stronger.

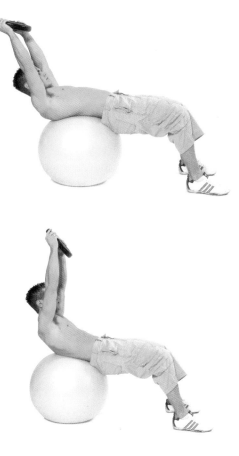

hanging leg raise*

target muscles: rectus abdominis (especially lower portion), transverse abdominis, hip flexors

starting position

1. Hang from a high bar with your hands shoulder-width apart. (You may use wrist or elbow straps for support.)
2. Your arms should be fully extended and your lower back slightly arched.

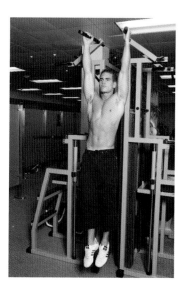

movement

1. Take your legs slightly behind your body.
2. Keeping your legs almost straight, exhale and raise them upwards as high as possible. Ideally, they should come just above the level of your hips. Focus on curling your hips towards your ribcage.
3. Hold for a count of two; then slowly return your legs to the starting position.

Make it easier: Bend your knees to reduce the resistance.

* If a chinning bar is not available, substitute Reverse Crunch (page 21) for this exercise.

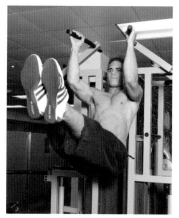

TIP

Do not swing your knees up or use the momentum of your legs – use the strength of your abdominals to move your hips and legs.

lateral exercise ball crunch

target muscles: internal and external obliques, rectus abdominis

starting position

1. Lie sideways over an exercise ball with your legs extended and your lower leg slightly bent behind the upper leg to give you enough stability.

2. Place your hands to the sides of your head.

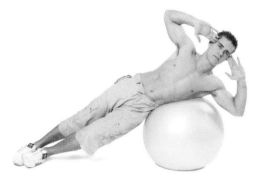

movement

1. Curl up your torso as high as you can. Make sure you do not move forwards or backwards.

2. Do the stated number of reps then switch sides.

> **TIP**
>
> This is quite a small movement so don't worry if you don't raise your torso very high. Focus on keeping your abs contracted.

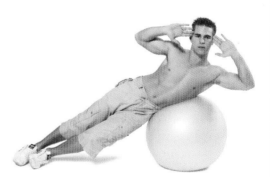

week 5

the goal

By week 5, you will have developed significant strength in your abdominal muscles. This week introduces some advanced variations of exercises that target the lower ab region and obliques. Again, do the first exercise in the superset immediately followed by the second exercise. Rest for 30 seconds before repeating the superset.

■ Perform the two exercises in the first superset. Rest for 30 seconds then repeat one more time.

■ Next, perform the second superset in the same manner, resting for 30 seconds between sets.

■ You should complete the workout in no more than nine minutes.

■ Perform each repetition with good technique (see exercise tips, pages 4–5).

exercise	sets	reps
Superset 1		
Plank with arms extended	2	1
Twisting hanging leg raise	2	10–12
Superset 2		
Exercise ball roll-out	2	10–12
Twisting exercise ball pull-in	2	12–15

plank with arms extended

target muscles: rectus abdominis, transverse abdominis

starting position

1. Lie face down with your hips and legs in contact with the floor, and your upper body raised and supported on your forearms.

2. Your elbows should be directly under your shoulders by the sides of your body, palms down.

movement

1. Lift your torso so that you assume a press-up position. You should be supporting your body weight on your hands and toes only. Keep your spine in neutral alignment – your head, back, hips and ankles should be in a straight line.

2. Hold for 60–120 seconds, then slowly lower yourself back to the starting position.

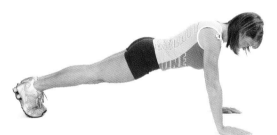

TIPS

• Keep your abs held in during the exercise to protect your back.

• Check your neck, torso and legs are in a straight line.

• Make sure you don't lift your bottom higher than your shoulders.

• Keep your shoulders pulled down and try to lengthen the distance between your shoulders and ears.

Make it harder: Perform this exercise with your feet on top of an exercise ball. Alternatively, you can perform this exercise on one leg. Once you are in the press-up position, raise one leg a few centimetres off the ground so you are balancing on your hands and the toes of one foot. Hold, then lower back to the starting position and repeat on the other leg.

twisting hanging leg raise*

target muscles: rectus abdominis (especially lower portion), obliques, hip flexors

starting position

1. Hang from a high bar with your hands shoulder-width apart and legs and feet together.
2. Your arms should be fully extended and your lower back slightly arched.

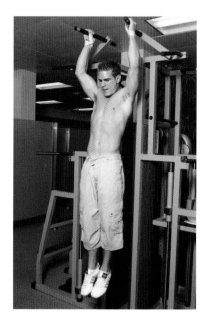

movement

1. Take your legs slightly behind your body.
2. Raise your knees as high as possible to one side – they should come just above the level of your hips. Curl your hips towards your ribcage.
3. Hold for a moment, then lower, alternating sides.

Make it harder: Complete all reps on one side before switching sides.

* If a chinning bar is not available, substitute Reverse Crunch (page 21) for this exercise.

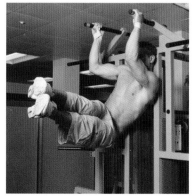

> **TIP**
>
> Avoid swinging your knees up – use the strength of your abdominals to move your hips and legs.

exercise ball roll-out

target muscles: rectus abdominis (lower), transverse abdominis

starting position

1. Kneel down in front of an exercise ball. Place your clasped hands on top of the ball with a slight bend in your elbows.

movement

1. Slowly roll the ball out in front of you until your hands, shoulders and hips make a straight line.
2. Hold for a moment then return to the starting position. Repeat.

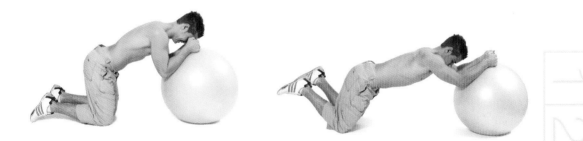

TIP

Don't bend at the hips. Keep your back as straight as possible throughout the movement.

twisting exercise ball pull-in

target muscles: rectus abdominis, obliques, transverse abdominis

starting position

1. Get into a push-up position, placing the lower part of your shins on top of an exercise ball.
2. Your head, back, hips and knees should be in a straight line.

movement

1. Slowly pull your left knee towards your right side instead of pulling your knees in straight.
2. Straighten your legs, rolling the ball back to the starting position. Then repeat to the other side.

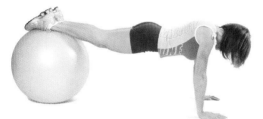 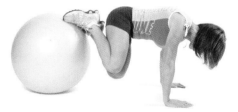

TIP

Keep your back straight throughout the movement.

week 6

the goal

During this final week, you will further challenge your abdominal muscles by performing three sets of each superset. This will feel tough but, remember, you have to push yourself hard if you want to get great results. This sixth workout targets all three areas of the abdominal region equally: upper, lower and side.

■ Perform the two exercises in the first superset. Rest for 30 seconds then repeat two more times.

■ Next, perform the second superset in the same manner, resting for 30 seconds between sets.

■ You should complete the workout in no more than nine minutes.

■ Perform each repetition with good technique (see exercise tips, page 4–5).

exercise	sets	reps
Superset 1		
Split-leg crunch	3	12–15
Lower body rotation on exercise ball	3	10–12
Superset 2		
Scissor kick	3	20–25
Exercise ball jackknife	3	10–15

split-leg crunch

target muscles: rectus abdominis, obliques, transverse abdominis

starting position

1. Lie flat on your back with your legs straight apart in the air.

movement

1. Raise your head and shoulders from the floor and reach to touch the toes of your right foot. Your lower back should remain on the floor.

2. Hold in this contracted position for a moment.

3. Let your body uncurl slowly back to the starting position. Repeat on alternate sides.

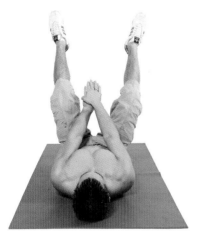
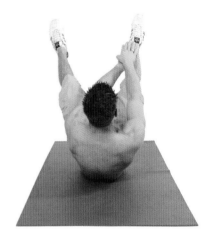

lower body rotation on exercise ball

target muscles: obliques, transverse abdominis

starting position

1. Get into a push-up position with your shins on top of an exercise ball, feet together. Keep your back and legs straight.

movement

1. Slowly rotate your lower body to the right, stopping before your right foot touches the floor. Return to the starting position.

2. Slowly rotate to the left, stopping before your left foot touches the floor.

> **TIP**
>
> Keep your head in line with your back throughout the exercise.

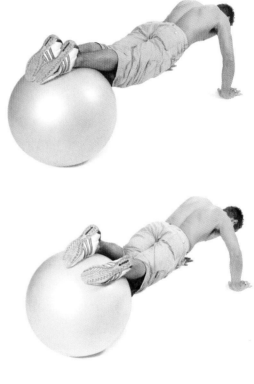

37

scissor kick

target muscles: rectus abdominis (lower part), transverse abdominis

starting position

1. Lie on your back with your arms extended by your sides, palms facing down and legs straight.

movement

1. Lift your legs a few centimetres from the floor. Then make up-and-down scissor movements as you raise each leg to about 45–60 degrees into the air and lower back to a few centimetres off the floor.

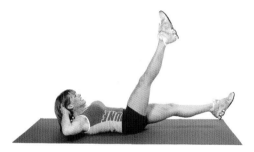
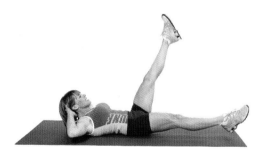

TIP

This movement is fairly rapid. Keep your back in neutral position, avoid arching, and keep your hips still throughout.

exercise ball jackknife

target muscles: rectus abdominis, transverse abdominis

starting position

1. Get into a push-up position, resting the lower part of your shins on top of an exercise ball.
2. Make sure your arms, back and legs are straight.

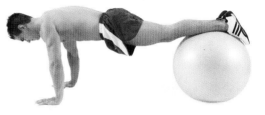

movement

1. Slowly pull your lower body in towards your hands, allowing the ball to roll forwards and raising your hips as high as you can.
2. Pause, contracting your abs hard, then roll the ball back to the starting position.

TIPS

- Keep the movement smooth and controlled.
- Roll the ball in as close to your hands as possible and tuck your chin in – your torso should be almost vertical.

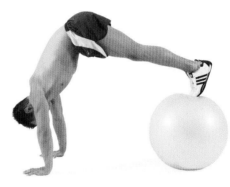

work your lower back

To support and stabilise your lower back you should include exercises that specifically target the lower back muscles (erector spinae) as well as your abs exercises. Aim to include two of the following exercises in your routine twice a week.

back extension

starting position

1. Lie face down on a mat or on the floor.
2. Place your hands by the sides of your head, elbows out to the sides. Alternatively, your arms may be placed on your back.

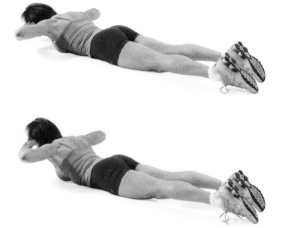

movement

1. Slowly raise your head, shoulders and upper chest from the floor. This will be just a short distance.
2. Pause for a count of two, then lower yourself slowly to the floor.

TIPS

- Keep your head facing downwards to the floor in line with your spine.
- Keep your legs relaxed on the floor – do not raise them.
- Only raise yourself as far as you feel comfortable.

back extension bench

starting position

1. Tuck your ankles underneath the pads and position your body so that your hips are resting on the middle pad, arms crossed in front of you.

movement

1. Raise your torso until you are parallel with the floor – do not lift higher than this.

2. Slowly bend forwards at the waist until you are almost at a right angle to the floor. Keep your back flat.

Make it harder: Place your hands along the sides of your head. Alternatively, if you are an advanced weight trainer, hold a small weight disc against your chest.

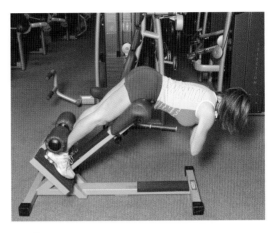

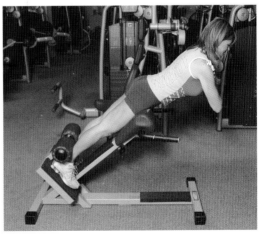

dorsal raise

starting position

1. Lie face down on a mat with your arms stretched out in front of you and your legs straight.

the movement

1. Slowly raise your right arm and your left leg, keeping them both straight. This will be just a short distance.

2. Hold for a count of two, then lower slowly to the floor. Repeat, raising the opposite arm and leg.

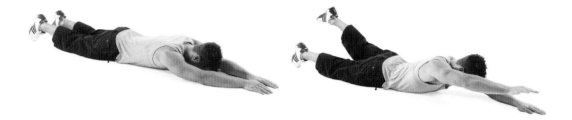

TIPS

• Keep your head facing downwards to the floor in line with your spine.

• Only lift as far as you feel comfortable.

back extension with exercise ball

starting position

1. Lie over the exercise ball, face down, keeping your hips halfway up the ball rather than balanced on top of it. Place your feet against a wall for support if you like.

2. Place your arms either crossed over your chest or by the sides of your head.

3. Keep your legs wide and straight out behind you.

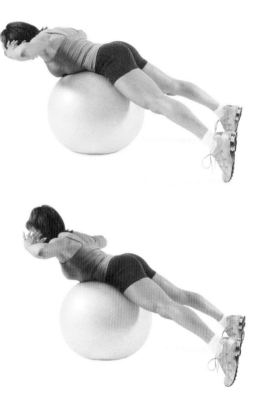

movement

1. Slowly raise your upper body in a straight line towards the ceiling.

2. Hold for a count of two, then slowly lower.

TIPS

- Do not arch your back.
- Keep your head in line with your spine.
- To make the movement harder, bring your legs closer together.

fat burning

To reveal those toned abs, you need to burn that layer of fat covering them up. This six-week cardiovascular (CV) workout is designed to produce the twin benefits of a leaner, more defined midsection and improved aerobic fitness and heart health.

burning calories

CV exercise burns calories not only when you're working out but also the rest of the time when you're not exercising. The table below shows you how many calories you can burn by performing a variety of different CV exercises.

CALORIE BURN OF VARIOUS ACTIVITIES *

Activity	Calories burned in 30 minutes
Running (jogging) 8.3 km/h or 5.2 mph	283
Running (fast) 12 km/h or 7.5 mph	438
Running (hard) 16 km/h or 10 mph	529
Cycling (moderate) 11.3 km/h or 7 mph	149
Cycling (fast) 16.1 km/h or 10 mph	225
Cycling (hard) 25.8 km/h or 16 mph	360
Swimming – crawl (moderate)	328
Swimming – crawl (fast)	599
Swimming – breast stroke	340
Swimming – back stroke	355
Elliptical trainer	390
Stair climber	270
Rowing machine	300
Walking (brisk)	168

* Based on a 70 kg person

cv workout guidelines

work out on an empty stomach

CV exercise performed first thing in the morning on an empty stomach burns more fat than at any other time. That's because insulin levels are at their lowest and glucagon levels are at their highest. This encourages your body to draw on its fat reserves for fuel. If you work out after eating your body will use this food for fuel instead. Exercising first thing in the morning also helps kick-start your metabolism so you'll burn more calories during the rest of the day.

do cv exercise and weights on separate days

If you want to build muscle mass as well as burn fat, try to do your CV workout on a different day from weights. Research suggests that overall calorie expenditure is greater if CV and weight-training exercise are done on separate days. That's because each time you train, your metabolism is boosted – so training on most days of the week will lead to faster fat loss. But if you have to do both in one session, complete your weight-training workout first when glycogen stores are high. Do it the other way round and you risk lower strength and muscle mass gains.

add intervals

Doing intervals – alternating short periods of high-intensity work with lower-intensity recovery periods – increases your calorie burn. It also helps you burn more calories afterwards. One US study found that interval training speeds up your metabolic rate for up to 18 hours after your workout. It also gets you fitter and strengthens your heart and lungs more than training at a steady pace. However, intervals are only suitable for those with a good level of fitness to start with. Beginners should build up basic fitness with steady-pace exercise first.

Intervals can be applied to any mode of CV exercise – running, cycling, stationary bike, stepping machine, elliptical trainer or any other cardio machine. Intersperse faster bursts of activity (e.g. increase the speed or the resistance of the machine) with more moderate recovery periods.

change your activity

Choosing the same CV activity each day can be boring and may also lead to a lower calorie burn as your body becomes more efficient in performing a movement over time. Try to choose a different CV activity each workout. Any of the following are suitable:

- running/treadmill
- fitness/power walking
- stepping machine/stair climber
- cycling/stationary bicycle
- swimming
- studio aerobic classes
- climbing machine
- elliptical training machine
- rowing machine.

use target heart rate training

Make sure you are working out at a safe and effective level by using target heart rate training. This is a measure of how hard you are working. First of all you need to estimate your maximal heart rate (MHR) by subtracting your age from 220. For example, if you are 30, your MHR would be 220 − 30 = 190 beats per minute (bpm). Consult the Heart Rate Training Guide overleaf to find out which zone you are training in. Each zone is basically a percentage of your MHR. Choose either the beginner, intermediate or advanced workout, depending on your experience level.

All three workouts burn fat and develop your fitness – although the high-intensity advanced workout is more efficient.

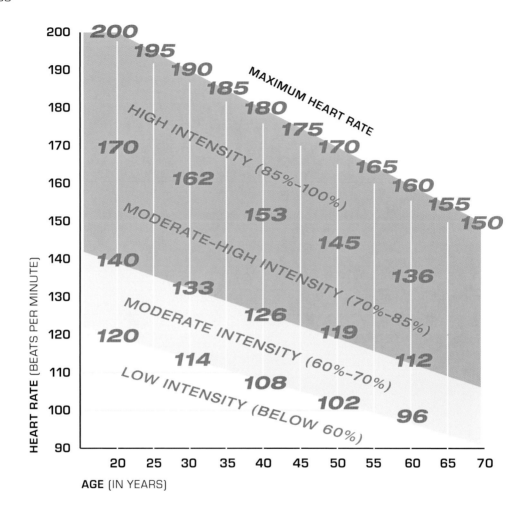

monitor your heart rate

The best way to monitor your heart rate during your workout is by using a heart rate monitor, or by taking your pulse manually. At regular intervals count your heart rate at your wrist or neck for 10 seconds and multiply that number by six (which gives you your heart rate in beats per minute). Check to see which target heart rate (THR) zone you are in (see above).

RATING OF PERCEIVED EXERTION (RPE)

At rest	1	Non-exercise HR
Light activity – sitting working	2	Non-exercise HR
Light activity – walking at leisurely pace	3	Non-exercise HR
Moderate activity – purposeful walking	4	Non-exercise HR
Moderate activity – brisk walking	5	Non-exercise HR
Somewhat hard activity – jogging	6	60% MHR
Hard activity – running, breathing harder	7	65–75% MHR
Very hard activity – running, conversation just possible	8	80% MHR
Very very hard activity – fast running, conversation difficult	9	85% MHR
Maximum effort – unable to speak	10	MHR

use perceived exertion to monitor intensity

If you don't have a heart rate monitor and find it difficult to work out your heart rate manually, you can use perceived exertion (PE) instead of THR to monitor the intensity of your CV workout (see Rating of Perceived Exertion opposite). This is a subjective rating of how hard you feel you are exercising. It is a 10-point scale ranging from 1 (no effort at all) to 10 (maximum effort). This system correlates closely with THR, so if you're working out at PE level 6 you are exercising at about 60 per cent of your MHR.

your cv workout

Your fat-burning CV workout consists of three parts: a warm-up (5 minutes), a CV session (20–40 minutes) and a cool-down (5 minutes).

The warm-up raises your body temperature, prepares your body for more strenuous exercise and reduces injury risk. The CV session should last for a minimum of 20 minutes. To make improvements over time you need to progressively challenge your system. This can be achieved by increasing the

BEGINNERS' STEADY PACE FAT-BURNER WORKOUT

Total exercise time = 30 minutes

Exercise time (minutes)	Stage	Intensity (THR)	Intensity (PE)
5	Warm-up	50%	5
20	Steady pace	60%	6
5	Cool-down	50%	5

INTERMEDIATE INTERVAL FAT-BURNER WORKOUT

Total exercise time = 34 minutes

Exercise time (minutes)	Stage	Intensity (THR)	Intensity (PE)
5	Warm-up	50%	5
2	Interval	70%	7
2	Recovery	60%	6
2	Interval	70%	7
2	Recovery	60%	6
2	Interval	70%	7
2	Recovery	60%	6
2	Interval	70%	7
2	Recovery	60%	6
2	Interval	70%	7
2	Recovery	60%	6
2	Interval	70%	7
2	Recovery	60%	6
5	Cool down	50%	5

ADVANCED INTERVAL FAT-BURNER WORKOUT

Total exercise time = 34 minutes

Exercise time (minutes)	Stage	Intensity (THR)	Intensity (PE)
5	Warm-up	50%	5
2	Interval	70%	7
2	Recovery	60%	6
1	Interval	80%	8–9
2	Recovery	60%	6
1	Interval	80%	8–9
2	Recovery	60%	6
1	Interval	80%	8–9
2	Recovery	60%	6
1	Interval	80%	8–9
2	Recovery	60%	6
1	Interval	80%	8–9
2	Recovery	60%	6
1	Interval	80%	8–9
2	Recovery	70%	7
2	Recovery	60%	6
5	Cool down	50%	5

number of times you work out per week, increasing your workout time, increasing the intensity (e.g. your speed or resistance of the machine) or adding more intervals.

The cool-down allows your body temperature, muscles and circulatory system time to return to normal. If you stop too quickly, you may feel dizzy and faint.

workout logs

Use the workout logs in this chapter to record your progress throughout the six-week workout programme.

day	workout	exercise	goal reps	actual reps
Monday	Abs workout	Pelvic tilt	15–20	Set 1: Set 2:
		Twisting exercise ball crunch	10–12	Set 1: Set 2:
		Side bridge	5	Set 1: Set 2:
		Crunch	12–20	Set 1: Set 2:
Tuesday	Beginner's fat-burner CV workout			
Wednesday	Abs workout	Pelvic tilt	15–20	Set 1: Set 2:
		Twisting exercise ball crunch	10–12	Set 1: Set 2:
		Side bridge	5	Set 1: Set 2:
		Crunch	12–20	Set 1: Set 2:
Thursday	Beginner's fat-burner CV workout			
Friday	Abs workout	Pelvic tilt	15–20	Set 1: Set 2:
		Twisting exercise ball crunch	10–12	Set 1: Set 2:
		Side bridge	5	Set 1: Set 2:
		Crunch	12–20	Set 1: Set 2:
Saturday	Beginner's fat-burner CV workout			
Sunday	Rest day			

week 1

week 2	day	workout	exercise	goal reps	actual reps
	Monday	Abs workout	Exercise ball crunch	12 – 15	Set 1: Set 2:
			Twisting crunch	10 – 12	Set 1: Set 2:
			Exercise ball pull-in	10	Set 1: Set 2:
			Plank	1	Set 1: Set 2:
	Tuesday	Beginner's fat-burner CV workout			
	Wednesday	Abs workout	Exercise ball crunch	12 – 15	Set 1: Set 2:
			Twisting crunch	10 – 12	Set 1: Set 2:
			Exercise ball pull-in	10	Set 1: Set 2:
			Plank	1	Set 1: Set 2:
	Thursday	Beginner's fat-burner CV workout			
	Friday	Abs workout	Exercise ball crunch	12 – 15	Set 1: Set 2:
			Twisting crunch	10 – 12	Set 1: Set 2:
			Exercise ball pull-in	10	Set 1: Set 2:
			Plank	1	Set 1: Set 2:
	Saturday	Beginner's fat-burner CV workout			
	Sunday	Rest day			

week 3

day	workout	exercise	goal reps	actual reps
Monday	Abs workout	Reverse crunch	10 – 12	Set 1: Set 2:
		Exercise ball jackknife	10 – 12	Set 1: Set 2:
		Side crunch	10	Set 1: Set 2:
		Lying alternate leg extensions	12 – 15	Set 1: Set 2:
Tuesday	Intermediate interval fat-burner CV workout			
Wednesday	Abs workout	Reverse crunch	10 – 12	Set 1: Set 2:
		Exercise ball jackknife	10 – 12	Set 1: Set 2
		Side crunch	10	Set 1: Set 2:
		Lying alternate leg extensions	12 – 15	Set 1: Set 2:
Thursday	Intermediate interval fat-burner CV workout			
Friday	Abs workout	Reverse crunch	10 – 12	Set 1: Set 2:
		Exercise ball jackknife	10 – 12	Set 1: Set 2:
		Side crunch	10	Set 1: Set 2:
		Lying alternate leg extensions	12 – 15	Set 1: Set 2:
Saturday	Intermediate interval fat-burner CV workout			
Sunday	Rest day			

week 4	day	workout	exercise	goal reps	actual reps
	Monday	Abs workout	Superset 1		
			Hip thrust	12–15	Set 1:
					Set 2:
			Pullover crunch on exercise ball	12–20	Set 1:
					Set 2:
			Superset 2		
			Hanging leg raise	10–12	Set 1:
					Set 2:
			Lateral exercise ball crunch	12–15	Set 1:
					Set 2:
	Tuesday	Intermediate interval fat-burner CV workout			
	Wednesday	Abs workout	Superset 1		
			Hip thrust	12–15	Set 1:
					Set 2:
			Pullover crunch on exercise ball	12–20	Set 1:
					Set 2:
			Superset 2		
			Hanging leg raise	10–12	Set 1:
					Set 2:
			Lateral exercise ball crunch	12–15	Set 1:
					Set 2:
	Thursday	Intermediate interval fat-burner CV workout			

Friday	Abs workout	Superset 1		
		Hip thrust	12 – 15	Set 1:
				Set 2:
		Pullover crunch on exercise ball	12 – 20	Set 1:
				Set 2:
		Superset 2		
		Hanging leg raise	10 – 12	Set 1:
				Set 2:
		Lateral exercise ball crunch	12 – 15	Set 1:
				Set 2:
Saturday	Intermediate interval fat-burner CV workout			
Sunday	Rest day			

	day	workout	exercise	goal reps	actual reps
week 5	Monday	Abs workout	Superset 1		
			One-leg plank with arms extended	1	Set 1: Set 2:
			Twisting hanging leg raise	10 – 12	Set 1: Set 2:
			Superset 2		
			Exercise ball roll-out	10 – 12	Set 1: Set 2:
			Twisting exercise ball pull-in	12 – 15	Set 1: Set 2:
	Tuesday	Advanced interval fat-burner CV workout			
	Wednesday	Abs workout	Superset 1		
			One-leg plank with arms extended	1	Set 1: Set 2:
			Twisting hanging leg raise	10 – 12	Set 1: Set 2:
			Superset 2		
			Exercise ball roll-out	10 – 12	Set 1: Set 2:
			Twisting exercise ball pull-in	12 – 15	Set 1: Set 2:
	Thursday	Advanced interval fat-burner CV workout			

Friday	Abs workout	Superset 1		
		One-leg plank with arms extended	1	Set 1: Set 2:
		Twisting hanging leg raise	10 – 12	Set 1: Set 2:
		Superset 2		
		Exercise ball roll-out	10 – 12	Set 1: Set 2:
		Twisting exercise ball pull-in	12 – 15	Set 1: Set 2:
Saturday	Advanced interval fat-burner CV workout			
Sunday	Rest day			

	day	workout	exercise	goal reps	actual reps
week 6	Monday	Abs workout	Superset 1		
			Split-leg crunch	12–15	Set 1: Set 2: Set 3:
			Lower body rotation on exercise ball	10–12	Set 1: Set 2: Set 3:
			Superset 2		
			Scissor kick	20–25	Set 1: Set 2: Set 3:
			Exercise ball jackknife	10–15	Set 1: Set 2: Set 3:
	Tuesday	Advanced interval fat-burner CV workout			
	Wednesday	Abs workout	Superset 1		
			Split-leg crunch	12–15	Set 1: Set 2: Set 3:
			Lower body rotation on exercise ball	10–12	Set 1: Set 2: Set 3:
			Superset 2		
			Scissor kick	20–25	Set 1: Set 2: Set 3:
			Exercise ball jackknife	10–15	Set 1: Set 2: Set 3:
	Thursday	Advanced interval fat-burner CV workout			

Friday	Abs workout	Superset 1		
		Split-leg crunch	12 – 15	Set 1: Set 2: Set 3:
		Lower body rotation on exercise ball	10 – 12	Set 1: Set 2: Set 3:
		Superset 2		
		Scissor kick	20 – 25	Set 1: Set 2: Set 3:
		Exercise ball jackknife	10 – 15	Set 1: Set 2: Set 3:
Saturday	Advanced interval fat-burner CV workout			
Sunday	Rest day			

nutrition

Direct ab work will tone and shape your muscles, and regular CV exercise will increase your body's daily calorie burn. But if you're serious about getting into shape, you need a smart eating plan too. A carefully planned diet will ensure you get enough nutrients without eating more calories than you need. Diet plays a big part when it comes to shedding those surplus pounds. But don't become obsessed with dieting or embark on weight-loss fads. Follow these diet tips and your abs will be ready to be revealed in six weeks!

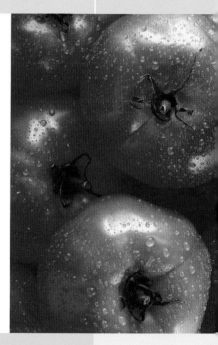

fab abs nutrition tips

do the maths

Half a kilo (1 lb) of fat equals roughly 3500 calories. In other words you can expect to lose 1 lb of body fat for every 3500 calories you omit from your diet and/or burn through exercise. This isn't as daunting as it sounds – lose 250 calories a day by foregoing two biscuits and drinking one less glass of wine, and burn an extra 250 calories through exercising.

practise portion control

Cut back your portion sizes by about 15 per cent. As a rule, the carbohydrate and protein portions should be no bigger than the size of your fist.

time your meals for greater fat-burning

If you want to burn more fat during your CV workout, exercise first thing in the morning on an empty stomach. Otherwise, try to avoid eating two to three hours before exercising. This will force your body to dip into its fat stores. If you eat before your workout, your muscles will burn more carbohydrate and less fat.

wait an hour after your workout before eating

After your workout, your body continues burning fat to replenish its fuel reserves. If you wait one hour before eating, this increases the residual fat-burning effect of exercise.

have a good breakfast

Eating breakfast kick-starts your metabolism. The calories will be used to fuel your daily activities and workouts instead of being stored as fat. Skipping breakfast increases the chances of snacking on high-calorie foods later in the day.

limit carbs

Eating too many carbs, especially at one sitting, provides your body with more than it needs for energy and glycogen stores. Anything left over will be stored as fat. The type of carbs you choose is important too. Refined, fibre-depleted carbs – white bread, white rice, biscuits and cakes – cause rapid surges in blood sugar levels, which in turn cause your body to release the hormone insulin. Too much insulin stimulates the appetite and encourages your body to store fat. Aim to eat no more than four to six servings of carbs per day, where a serving is about the size of your fist or two slices of bread.

Choose unrefined, fibre-rich carbs that provide a slow energy release: fruit, vegetables, whole-grain bread, pasta, rice, potatoes and sweetcorn.

EASY CALORIE SWAPS

REPLACE	WITH	CALORIES SAVED
1 oz mild Cheddar cheese	½ oz very strong Cheddar cheese	70–100
Oil for cooking	Oil spray	120/tablespoon
Pain au chocolate	2 slices wholemeal toast with Marmite	100
Buttered/sweet popcorn	Salted popcorn	95 per 75 g portion
Crisps	Twiglets	50 per 25 g bag
2 chocolate biscuits	2 rice cakes with jam	60
Shop-bought meat lasagne	Vegetable lasagne	173 per 420 g portion
Chicken korma	Chicken tikka	230 per 350 g portion
Chocolate bar	Breakfast or cereal bar	150
Cola	Water	136 per 330 ml can
Creamy fruit yoghurt	Very low-fat yoghurt	119 per 150 g pot
1 pint lager	1 glass dry white wine	74
1 glass fruit juice	1 glass half-and-half juice and water	50

lean on protein

When you take in fewer calories you risk losing muscle mass, so you need to up your protein intake. The best way to do this is to include a portion of protein with each meal. Good sources are fish, chicken, turkey, low-fat cheese, eggs, Quorn, soya, beans, lentils or yoghurt. Experts recommend increasing your protein intake by about 0.2 g per kilo of body weight. That's an extra 14 g daily for someone weighing 70 kg, equivalent to 2 eggs or half a chicken breast. Studies have also shown that protein blunts your appetite more than carbohydrate or fat. If you skimp on protein you could find yourself still hungry after you've eaten.

eat more healthy fats

Very low-fat diets are bad for your health and won't necessarily make you lose weight. A moderate intake of healthy fats improves appetite control and helps you burn body fat. Fats to avoid are:

Saturated (animal) fats (fatty meat, full-fat dairy products, butter and any products made with palm oil or palm kernel oil);

Processed (hydrogenated) fats (margarine, low-fat spreads, pastries, pies, biscuits, cereal bars, breakfast bars, cakes and bakery products, ice cream, desserts and puddings).

Heart-healthy alternatives are:

Monounsaturated fats (olive oil, nuts, seeds, avocados and rapeseed oil);

Essential omega-3 fats (oily fish, walnuts, omega-3-rich oils and omega-3-rich eggs).

Studies show that rebalancing your fat intake this way helps speed weight loss, improves oxygen delivery to your cells, boosts your metabolism and lowers your blood cholesterol.

eat 5-6 small meals a day

Never skip meals, no matter how busy you are. Leaving gaps longer than four hours between meals not only saps your energy but also triggers muscle loss as your body turns to protein for fuel. Eat five or six small meals spread over the day – breakfast, lunch and evening meal with two or three healthy snacks in between. Small regular meals keep your metabolism revved (burning 10 per

RECOMMENDED DAILY PORTIONS OF EACH FOOD GROUP

Food group	Number of portions each day	Food	Portion size
Vegetables	3–5	**1 portion = 80 g** Broccoli, cauliflower	2–3 spears/florets
		Carrots	1 carrot
		Peas	3 tablespoons
		Other vegetables	3 tablespoons
		Tomatoes	5 cherry tomatoes
Fruit	2–4	**1 portion = 80 g** Apple, pear, peach, banana	1 medium fruit
		Plum, kiwi fruit, satsuma	1–2 fruit
		Strawberries	8–10
		Grapes	12–16
		Tinned fruit	3 tablespoons
		Fruit juice	1 medium glass
Grains and potatoes	4–6	Bread	2 slices
		Rolls/muffins	1 roll
		Pasta or rice	6 tablespoons
		Breakfast cereal	1 bowl

		Potatoes, sweet potatoes, yams	Size of your fist
Calcium-rich foods	2–4	Milk (dairy or calcium-fortified soya milk)	1 medium cup
		Cheese	Size of 4 dice
		Tofu	Size of 4 dice
		Tinned sardines	1–2 tablespoons
		Yoghurt/fromage frais	1 pot
Protein-rich foods	2–4	Lean meat	1–2 slices (40–80 g)
		Poultry	2 medium slices/1 breast
		Fish	1 fillet
		Eggs	2
		Lentils/beans	Size of your palm
		Tofu/soya burger or sausage	1–2
Healthy fats and oils	1	Nuts and seeds	1 heaped tablespoon
		Seed oils, nut oils	1 tablespoon
		Avocado	Half
		Oily fish*	Deck of cards

*Oily fish is very rich in essential fats so just 1 portion a week would cover your need

cent more calories for two hours after eating) so you burn off more calories each day.

watch those evening nibbles

Forget big evening meals if you want to get and stay lean! Overeat in the evening and most of the calories will be stored as body fat. Aim to eat the majority of your daily calories during the morning and afternoon – spread over breakfast, lunch and two or three snacks – as this will up your metabolic rate and promote fat-burning.

veg out

Vegetables help you feel full without boosting your daily calorie intake. Three generous sprigs of broccoli contain just 45 calories, about the same as a nibble (one square) of chocolate. Aim for three to five portions of veg a day, and a minimum of two portions of fruit. Go easy on carbs and fat in the evening, and fill up instead with plenty of vegetables and fresh fruit. Try replacing half of your usual portion of pasta (or whatever) with a cupful of carrots, broccoli, green beans or cauliflower. That way you won't feel like you're eating less.

don't go for the quick fix

Quick-fix snacks and nibbles are full of sugar, saturated fat and salt – all great energy-sappers. Worse, they encourage you to overeat as they have poor filling power and don't make much of a dent on your appetite. Instead, plan your diet around nutritious low-GI (slow release) foods, which provide vitamins, minerals and fibre, and more stable blood sugar levels.

count those alcohol calories too

Alcohol can encourage fat storage. It's high in calories, puts undue stress on the liver and can hinder your recovery after intense workouts. Stick to safe intakes – fewer than 21 weekly units for men and fewer than 14 for women (1 unit is half a pint of ordinary beer or a small glass (125 ml) of wine).

balance your blood sugar levels

Include low-GI foods in your meals to give a slow blood sugar release. Good options include oats, beans, lentils, vegetables and fruit. Combine your carbs with lean protein or healthy fats for a sustained energy release. Try jacket potatoes with tuna or a drizzle of olive oil.

balance your diet

Aim to include the number of daily portions of each food group suggested on pages 66–67.

menu plans

Each day, you should have three meals (breakfast, lunch and an evening meal) and two or three healthy snacks. Here are some suggestions for the first week of the Fab Abs programme.

day 1 menu plan

breakfast

Porridge with Raisins
Porridge made with 45 g oats and 200 ml skimmed or
semi-skimmed milk, topped with 2 tablespoons (30 ml) raisins

lunch

Turkey and Rocket Baguette
100 g French bread split and filled with 40 g sliced cooked turkey,
2 teaspoons reduced-fat mayonnaise, a handful of rocket and
tomato slices
1 portion of fresh fruit

evening meal

Pan-fried Tuna with Spinach and Pine Nuts
85 g tinned pineapple or peaches

snacks

1 pot low-fat fruit yoghurt
1 slice wholemeal toast with 1 teaspoon olive oil spread and
2 teaspoons jam

pan-fried tuna with spinach and pine nuts

■ Heat a non-stick pan until very hot. Brush a 150 g tuna steak with olive oil and place in the pan. Cook for 2 minutes on each side, until just charred. Remove from the heat.

■ Wash 125 g of fresh spinach and place in a saucepan. If using ready-washed spinach, add 1–2 tablespoons of water. Cook over a gentle heat until wilted. Drain off any excess liquid, return to the pan and add 1 teaspoon (5 ml) olive oil spread, 1 tablespoon (15 ml) pine nuts and a little salt and pepper to taste. Spoon onto a serving plate and top with the tuna and a lemon wedge. Accompany with 1 medium jacket potato (125 g cooked weight).

day 2 menu plan

breakfast

Muesli with Fruit
40 g muesli (homemade or bought) with 125 ml skimmed or
semi-skimmed milk and 125 g strawberries or sliced peaches

lunch

Spinach, Rocket and Avocado Salad
Mix together a handful of spinach and rocket leaves in a large bowl.
Combine with half an avocado (thinly sliced), 1 tablespoon (15 ml) of
nuts (e.g. cashews, walnuts, peanuts) and 1 tablespoon (15 ml)
balsamic vinegar
1 small wholemeal roll with 2 teaspoons (10 ml) olive oil spread

evening meal

Chicken and Vegetable Kebabs with Yoghurt Sauce
1 portion of fresh fruit

snacks

1 apple and 1 large banana
2 crispbreads with 2 teaspoons peanut butter

chicken and vegetable kebabs with yoghurt sauce

- First, make the sauce by combining 2 tablespoons (30 ml) plain yoghurt with 1 small garlic clove (crushed), 1 tablespoon (15 ml) lemon juice and ½ teaspoon (2.5 ml) chopped mint. Cut a large, boned chicken breast into chunks, then coat with the yoghurt mixture. Leave to marinate in the fridge for an hour.

- Preheat the grill. Thread alternate pieces of chicken, cherry tomatoes, courgette slices and yellow pepper onto 2 skewers and grill for about 15 minutes, turning and basting with some of the remaining marinade, until cooked. Heat and serve the remaining marinade as an accompanying sauce. Serve with 3 heaped tablespoons of cooked rice (150 g cooked weight).

Vegetarian: Substitute 100 g tofu for the chicken.

day 3 menu plan

breakfast

Fruit 'n' Yoghurt
Place 85–125 g fresh fruit – e.g. chopped mango, sliced bananas, strawberries, raspberries or blueberries – in a bowl and spoon over 150 g natural bio yoghurt. Drizzle over 1–2 level teaspoons (5–10 ml) honey

lunch

Carrot Soup with Crusty Bread
300 ml fresh carrot soup with coriander (bought or homemade) accompanied by 1 large slice of crusty wholemeal bread with a little olive oil spread. Scatter over 2 tablespoons (30ml) grated cheddar cheese.

evening meal

Grilled Chicken with Pasta
50 g low-fat frozen yoghurt dessert topped with 85 g sliced strawberries, raspberries or blueberries.

snacks

Small banana and 4 dried apricots
1 small wholemeal roll with 1 teaspoon spread and Marmite

grilled chicken with pasta

■ 125 g chicken breast, brushed with olive oil and grilled, served with 3 heaped tablespoons (150 g cooked weight) pasta (preferably whole wheat) and 225 g steamed vegetables (e.g. carrots, broccoli, courgettes, green beans).

Vegetarian: Substitute a grilled bean burger for the chicken.

day 4 menu plan

breakfast

Toasted English Muffin with Marmalade
1 toasted wholemeal English muffin with 1 teaspoon olive oil spread
and 2 level teaspoons (2 x 5 ml) marmalade
1 portion of fresh fruit

lunch

Bagel with Rocket, Pesto and Paprika Chicken
1 portion fresh fruit

evening meal

Grilled Fish with Roasted Vegetables

snacks

$\frac{1}{2}$ English muffin with 1 teaspoon spread; 1 small piece of fruit
(e.g. satsuma)
1 banana mixed with 2 tablespoons low-fat plain yoghurt

bagel with rocket, pesto and paprika chicken

■ Place 85 g chicken fillets in a dish and toss with $\frac{1}{2}$ – 1 teaspoon (2.5 – 5 ml) dried basil or thyme, a pinch of paprika and 1 teaspoon (5 ml) olive oil. Sauté in a non-stick pan over a moderate heat until cooked.

■ Spread half a bagel with 1 teaspoon (5 ml) red pesto and top with a handful of rocket and a few slices of tomato. Slice the chicken into thin strips and arrange over the bagels. Scatter over freshly ground black pepper.

grilled fish with roasted vegetables

■ 120 g grilled white fish fillet (e.g. cod or haddock) OR 3 tablespoons (100 g) tinned beans (e.g. pinto beans, chickpeas, red kidney beans) accompanied by 225 g vegetables (e.g. courgettes, peppers, onions, aubergines, tomatoes) tossed in 1 tablespoon olive oil, 1 crushed garlic clove and rosemary sprigs and roasted at 200°C/400°F/Gas Mark 6 for about 30 minutes. Serve with one medium jacket potato (125 g cooked weight) with a dab of olive oil spread.

day 5 menu plan

breakfast

Toast and Honey (or Jam)
A slice of wholemeal toast with 2 teaspoons (10 ml) olive oil spread
and 2 teaspoons (10 ml) honey (or jam)
1 portion of fresh fruit

lunch

Filled Jacket Potato with Salad
1 medium jacket potato (125 g cooked weight) topped with 45 g
tuna tinned in spring water (drained) mixed with 1 tablespoon
sweetcorn and 2 teaspoons (10 ml) reduced-fat mayonnaise
A large mixed salad with 1 tablespoon olive oil dressing
Vegetarian: Substitute 1–2 tablespoons (15–30 ml) hummus for
the tuna
1 portion of fresh fruit

evening meal

Chicken, Red Pepper and Tarragon Rice Salad
1 pot (150 g) natural yoghurt mixed with 3 chopped dried apricots

snacks

1 piece of fresh fruit with 1 tablespoon nuts or seeds
1 small bowl (25 g) bran flakes/cornflakes with 150 ml
skimmed milk

chicken, red pepper and tarragon rice salad

- First, make the dressing by mixing together 1 tablespoon olive oil, the juice of half a lemon, ½ teaspoon Dijon mustard, half a crushed garlic clove and 1 tablespoon chopped tarragon.

- Place the following ingredients in a large bowl: 3 tablespoons cooked brown or white rice (150 g cooked weight), half a red pepper (thinly sliced), 8 cherry tomatoes and 60 g cooked chicken. Pour over the dressing and mix thoroughly.

Vegetarian: Use 85 g tinned beans (e.g. red kidney beans) instead of the chicken.

day 6 menu plan

breakfast

Fresh Fruit Smoothie
Place in the goblet of a smoothie maker, blender or food processor 225 g of mixed fresh fruit (e.g. nectarine, melon, banana, oranges, peaches, strawberries, kiwi fruit or mango), 200 ml fruit juice and a handful of ice cubes. Process for about 45 seconds, until smooth. Serve immediately.

lunch

Open Sandwich with Guacamole and Tomatoes
Top a thick slice of bread with 1 heaped tablespoon (45 g) guacamole (homemade or bought), thin slices of tomato and a thinly sliced red pepper. Accompany with a mixed leaf salad with a drizzle of olive oil dressing.
1 pot (150 ml) natural yoghurt mixed with 1 tablespoon (15 g) dried fruit (e.g. raisins or chopped apricots)

evening meal

Stir-fried Chicken with Broccoli

snacks

5 Brazil nuts or walnuts
1 hot cross bun

stir-fried chicken with broccoli

■ Stir-fry 85 g chicken breast (cut into strips) for 2–3 minutes in 1 tablespoon (15 ml) olive oil. Remove from the pan. Meanwhile add half a small chopped onion, 60 g broccoli florets and a little grated ginger and stir-fry for 1 minute. Return the chicken to the pan and heat through.

■ Serve with 4 tablespoons cooked noodles (230 g cooked weight) and scatter over 1 tablespoon (15 g) cashew nuts.

Vegetarian: Use 85 g tofu instead of the chicken.

day 7 menu plan

breakfast

Cereal with Fruit
45 g bran flakes (or other bran/wholegrain cereal) topped with 1 portion of fresh fruit (e.g. sliced banana, apricots, strawberries or grated apple) served with 125 ml skimmed or semi-skimmed milk

lunch

Tuna and Butter Bean Salad
1 portion of fresh fruit

evening meal

Lean Home-made Turkey Burger on Ciabatta Bread
1 bowlful (125 g) fresh fruit salad (homemade or bought)

snacks

1 (200 ml) yoghurt drink
1 wholemeal cracker with 1 tablespoon hummus and carrot, cucumber and celery sticks

tuna and butter bean salad

- Arrange 50 g of watercress (or other salad leaves) on a plate. Spoon 100 g tuna (tinned in spring water, drained and rinsed) on top, breaking it up as you go. Scatter over 100 g (approximately a quarter of a 410 g can) butter beans.

- Pour over 1 tablespoon of dressing made by mixing 1 tablespoon of olive oil, a squeeze of lemon juice and a little salt and pepper.

Vegetarian: Use 100 g of another bean variety (e.g. red kidney beans or flageolet beans) instead of the tuna.

lean home-made turkey burger on ciabatta bread

■ This makes 4 servings. Mix together 225 g lean minced turkey (or other meat), half a small chopped onion, 1 crushed garlic clove, 1 teaspoon (5 ml) chopped fresh parsley and a little salt and black pepper. Form into 4 neat burger shapes. Place on a baking tray, spray with oil and cook under a hot grill for 10–15 minutes, turning frequently.

■ Meanwhile, toast 4 slices of ciabatta bread. Lay green salad leaves on the toasted bread then top with a burger. A burger counts as 1 serving. Accompany with a large mixed salad with 1 tablespoon olive oil dressing.

Vegetarian: Substitute a nut burger (homemade or bought) for the turkey burger.

more ideas for meals and snacks

breakfast

Wholemeal toast with honey and a carton of yoghurt

Porridge made with skimmed milk and some raisins

Muesli, Weetabix, Shreddies or Shredded Wheat with skimmed milk and fresh fruit

Fresh fruit salad with yoghurt and sunflower seeds

Toasted bagel or muffin with fresh fruit

mid-morning snack

Fresh fruit

Homemade or bought smoothie

Handful of cashews or peanuts and raisins

Handful of dried fruit – raisins, apricots, dates, blueberries, mango

lunch

Pasta with tomato and vegetable sauce and grated cheese

Wholemeal sandwich with chicken, tuna, peanut butter or cottage cheese, and salad

Jacket potato with baked beans, tuna or ratatouille and salad

Grilled fish, chicken or cooked beans with large salad

Lentil, chicken or bean soup with wholemeal roll and salad

Wholemeal roll, pitta bread or wrap filled with turkey and salad

Pasta with tuna and sweetcorn

Baked beans on toast and salad

Hummus with vegetable crudités and avocado slices

Smoked salmon with salad

mid-afternoon snack

Rice cakes with peanut butter

Fresh fruit with yoghurt

Milkshake made with skimmed milk, fresh fruit and yoghurt

Mixed sunflower and sesame seeds and raisins

evening meal

Grilled or baked fish with jacket potato (optional) and steamed vegetables

Prawn or marinated tofu and vegetable stir-fry with wholegrain rice (optional)

Grilled chicken or turkey breast with salad and new potatoes (optional)

Turkey, lentil or Quorn and vegetable curry

Chicken or vegetable paella

Mixed-bean chilli with salad

Lentil and vegetable soup

Bolognese made with turkey or beef mince or Quorn with pasta (optional) and vegetables

Kebabs made with lean meat or marinated tofu, peppers, courgettes, mushrooms and tomatoes, and wholegrain rice (optional)

Grilled sardines (or other oily fish) with grilled Mediterranean vegetables

maintenance

Congratulations on reaching the end of this six-week programme! Hopefully, you have now achieved your initial goals and are pleased with your results.

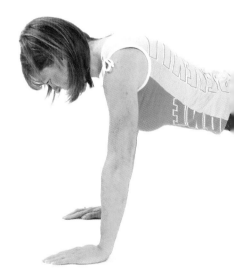

moving on

This six-week programme has introduced you to new exercises, and helped you to establish healthier diet and activity habits. But the programme doesn't end just because the book does. Give yourself a short break from the plan – I suggest a week – then decide on your next goal. If you need to shed more fat, you can repeat the programme. Alternatively, you can incorporate many of the positive elements of this programme into a longer-term plan to maintain your fab abs and your overall fitness.

Stick to the following principles.

■ Aim to complete three CV workouts for a minimum of 20 minutes each week.

■ Vary your activity as often as possible to increase your calorie burn, boost your motivation and reduce injury risk.

■ Monitor your heart rate or use your RPE to ensure you are continually challenging your body – make sure that you push yourself hard enough every workout.

■ Aim to complete an abs workout at least twice a week. Choose any of the six workouts in this book and try to vary the exercises you do as much as possible.

■ Avoid working your abs hard two days in a row. Try to leave at least one day between workouts.

■ Reread 'Exercise Tips' on pages 4–5, to make sure you don't lapse into bad habits.

■ Always stand, sit and walk with good posture – see page 4.

■ Continue to eat smart – reread the tips in Chapter 5, and use the diet plans and meal suggestions for the basis of your eating plan

Best wishes and good luck!

index